S0-DZC-650

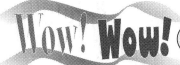 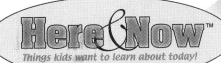

Wow! Wow! **Here Now™** *Things kids want to learn about today!* Wow! Wow!

Flip
through
the pages
to see the
couple
kiss!

The Here & Now Reproducible Book of

The 25 Most Asked Questions About Sex

Questions Kids Ask Parents and Teachers Today...and the Honest Answers!

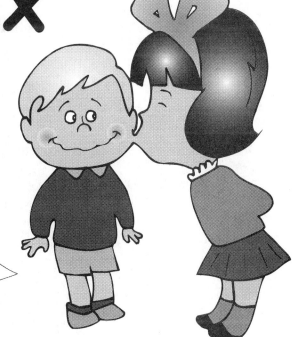

by Carole Marsh
author of Smart Sex Stuff for Kids 7-17

REPRODUCIBLE

GALL**O**PADE™ INTERNATIONAL

Editorial Assistant: Billie Walburn   Graphic Artist: Cecil Anderson

For additional information, go to our website at **www.gallopade.com**.

 1...

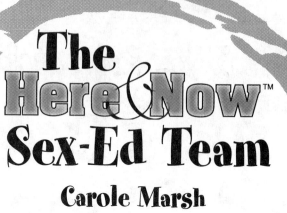

The Here & Now™ Sex-Ed Team

Carole Marsh
Billie Walburn
Cecil Anderson
Victoria DeJoy
Chad Beard

Published by

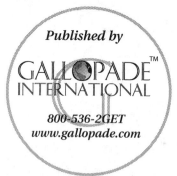

GALLOPADE™ INTERNATIONAL

800-536-2GET
www.gallopade.com

Gallopade is proud to be a member of these educational organizations and associations:

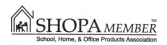

SHOPA MEMBER™
School, Home, & Office Products Association

NSSEA

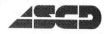

ASCD

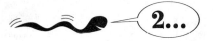

2...

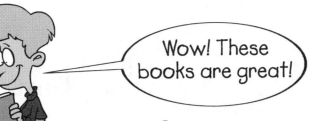

Other Here & Now™ Books

Classroom Cooking:
E-Z, Fun, Healthy, Educational, Historical Things to Cook Up Right in the Classroom

George W. Bush:
America's Newest President, and His White House Family

Good Magic, Spells, Potions, and More:
from History, Literature, and Make-Believe

America's Important Neighbors:
Canada, Mexico, and Cuba

The Budding Genius Book:
Activities on Latin, Chess, Bridge, Shakespeare, Physics, and More for Pre-Schoolers, Kindergarteners, and Early Elementary Students

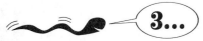

3...

Table of Contents

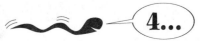

A Word From The Author

Dear Parents and Teachers,

Dad says, "Go ask Mom." Mom says, "Go ask Dad." Teachers say (usually silently), "Why are you asking me?!" Yes, most everyone wishes those kids-ask-the-darndest-things questions about sex would just go away. No such luck!

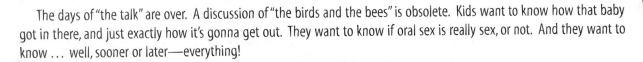

The thing that really startles us these days is the young age at which the questions begin … and how provocative some of the questions can be. But why are we surprised? The media so bombards us with sexual images, the news is so blatant, that kids who hear a new word, term, or phrase, can't help but ask, "What does that mean?"

If they're old enough to ask, they're old enough to get a respectful answer. You can anticipate many of these questions by monitoring the media yourself. You can delay some of the questions by taking pediatricians' recent advice to heart to limit how many sexual images (newspapers, magazines, videos, commercials, etc.) your child sees. However, you're never gonna avoid the questions, so get ready!

The days of "the talk" are over. A discussion of "the birds and the bees" is obsolete. Kids want to know how that baby got in there, and just exactly how it's gonna get out. They want to know if oral sex is really sex, or not. And they want to know … well, sooner or later—everything!

TIPS:
- Answer them honestly.
- Be accurate.
- Use real words. (A penis is a penis, not a peanut or a hot dog or a weenie.)
- Be respectful.
- Don't preach or lecture.
- Keep it brief; they want an answer, not an encyclopedia of reproductive plumbing!
- Use tools: books, articles, etc.
- Have a sense of humor.
- Learn more about sex yourself—there are some funny animal/insect/fish sex facts in this book that are fascinating!

Above all, plan to get past those body part building block words and the basic reproductive plumbing explanations, so you can move on to the really important stuff: relationships and responsibilities. We all are sexual beings our entire lives; kids want and need you as a partner in their ongoing search for the meaning of this facet of their lives. You can do it!

Carole Marsh

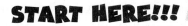

START HERE!!!

5…

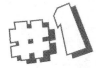

#1

While parents have always said they wanted kids to learn about sex in the home, current studies show kids are doing just that—having sex at home after school, while their parents are still at work!!

Hor(mones) Today—Gone Tomorrow!

Sooner or later, boys and girls get very interested in girls and boys. It may not be sexual at first. But as feelings change, a great interest in another person's body and wanting to have sexual relations with him or her is a common—and oftentimes, *very* intense feeling. So, why is a kid's body so interested in sex when they're still far too young to cope with the problems and responsibilities sex can create?

It's those "horny" hormones at work again! Peer pressure, curiosity, strong sex urges, "sexy" tv, movies, record lyrics, friends who swear they have sex, someone who says, "*If you really love me...*", or feeling like they're the last virgin on earth may *egg* kids into having sex—even when they know they're too young.

Q: Where do babies come from?

A: EXACTLY how does a girl get pregnant? Let's be very specific:

When the male's penis is inserted through the female's vulva into her vagina, semen comes out of his penis. Semen carries sperm that travel up though the vagina to meet an egg held in the female's reproductive organs. The sperm reach the egg. The egg is fertilized. The female becomes pregnant with a baby. Approximately nine months later, the baby travels down through the female's body and is delivered through the vagina.

Don't kid yourself–sperm are pretty squiggly stuff! If semen leaks out of the penis near the vaginal opening, those squirmy sperm can still sometimes find their way into the vagina. How many sperm are in a drop of semen? *Millions!* How many sperm does it take to fertilize an egg? One!

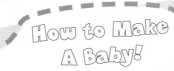

How to Make A Baby!

INGREDIENTS: 1 Egg/1 Sperm
UTENSILS: 1 Penis/1 Vagina

TO PREPARE: Take 1 erect penis and place in 1 vagina. Ejaculate. One sperm will fertilize one egg. (Discard other 999,999 sperm.) Let fertilized egg bake in warm uterus for nine months. When baby is done, it will eject from the vagina. Wrap in blanket to keep warm.
Serves: 2 for 18 years/**Cost per serving**: $100,000

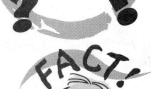

Discussion Questions?

How does a baby change lives? Do the changes affect the boy, too?

FACT!

Can I get pregnant the first time I have sex? **YES!**
You can even get pregnant using condoms or taking the Pill.

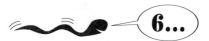

6...

#2

Today, it appears girls are entering puberty at a younger age. Some girls may have their first period as early as age 8! Some researchers believe trace elements of estrogen in our water supply may be a factor in early menses.

Q: Is a period more than a punctuation mark?

You're lucky to be able to get some honest and accurate, and timely information. Having your first period is evidence you're becoming a woman and your body's preparing to be able to have a child, when and if that time ever comes. Since that's how we all get here in the first place, and that's what keeps life on earth "keeping on"—it's no wonder that everyone in most every country and culture considers this first period a big deal!

A: A period is just one part of your reproductive cycle...

...a very ordinary and normal event that takes place over and over. The entire menstrual cycle is the repeated preparation of a woman's body to reproduce another human being *(a little one, called a baby, of course)—and* here's how the cycle goes:

● The pituitary gland at the base of your brain scoots out hormones that travel through the blood stream to the ovaries. The hormones cause one of the ovaries to begin ripening an egg. Don't worry, this egg's not as big as a chicken egg or anything—it's almost invisible! When a girl is born, her ovaries contain about 400,000 eggs. Only about 400 of these will ever be released from the ovaries. We really aren't sure why you have so many "spares." Usually an egg is ripened in one ovary one month and the other ovary (you have two), the next. After an egg has ripened, it comes out of the ovary. This is called ovulation. Most girls never feel this happen.

● This menstrual or reproductive cycle takes about 28 days altogether. Ovulation occurs about halfway through the cycle, or about 14 days after each period, once you begin to have them. The egg goes into the Fallopian tube nearest it and travels down to the uterus. Even in this tube, the egg can be fertilized. An egg gets fertilized through sexual intercourse. If the egg is fertilized, the woman becomes pregnant—which means she's going to have a baby!

● If the egg is not fertilized *(which of course, it can't be if you don't have sexual intercourse),* it and the lining shed from the uterus through the vagina. This is your period. The lining in the uterus is mostly made of blood. So, what comes out of the vagina is a small amount of bloody fluid. "Period" blood is blood that you don't need. It's only a small amount—about half a cup. It takes several days for this bloody discharge to drain out of your vagina. This is called the menstrual flow. This flow starts very slowly, just a trickle. Then it increases for a couple of days. Next, it tapers off until it stops completely.

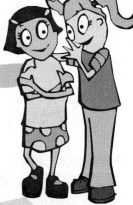

! Class Discussion !

Talk about what a period isn't! It isn't a "curse" or anything awful or terrible. It isn't something to be ashamed of or embarrassed about! It isn't something somebody knows you're having by looking at you. You're not sick. It's not dirty.

FACT!
Fact or Fiction—

Women might have thought it was best to skip school, or work, go to bed, or otherwise give in to their period. But these days, girls and women keep right on going: to school, to work, to the Olympics, even into space!

It's True!

When you first begin to menstruate (have your periods), they may be irregular. One time the flow might be heavy and last for more than a week. The next time, it might be light and just last for a few days. Once the hormones which are causing the periods get regular, your periods will settle down into a very familiar pattern, which you can pretty much count on to be "normal" for you.

#3 Many teens are deciding to wait to have sex. A lot of smart kids have decided that the hassle and worry over getting caught, pregnant, AIDS or another disease—just isn't worth it. One successful weapon in the battle against kids having sex is the "virginity pledge." Recent government-sponsored research indicates on the average, kids who took "the pledge" delayed having sex about one-third longer—18 months or more! To be effective, young pledgers must feel the size of the pledge group is not too big or too small—they need to feel part of a special group. They are special!

Q: What is a virgin?

A: A person who has not had sexual intercourse.

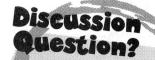

Discussion Question?

What are the pros and cons of being a virgin?

One thing we can teach even a young child about is their body. After all it's theirs—for life. Their body is theirs to take care of, keep to themselves, or later share—it's all up to them.

Many teens have the confidence and self-esteem to choose abstinence until marriage. They believe it's the right thing to do according to their morals, and the values they've been taught!

TAKE RESPONSIBILITY FOR YOUR OWN SEX LIFE!

I'd like to say that your sex life matters most to your parents, your teachers, the government, the health department, your girlfriend or boyfriend, or someone else, but it doesn't. It matters most to you. You are the one who will reap the benefits of abstinence. You are the one who will suffer the effects of premarital sex. Do you really think your friends will come to the labor room on prom night or pay part of your child support? *Riiiiiight!*

Just don't have sex with anyone until you either get married, or, choose someone to have a very, very long-term relationship with (this does NOT mean 6 weeks!). Just don't. Plan on it. Decide it. Choose it. And then don't change your mind, and don't let anyone else.

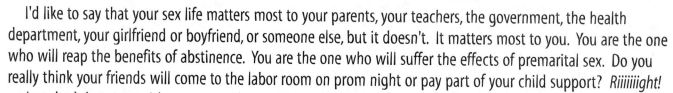

FACT! Virgin is NOT a dirty word! FACT!

Abstain from sex because you're selfish. This is a good kind of selfish—the best kind of selfish. It's your body and you don't have to share it with anyone until you are ready. You have a lot of things you want that body to do: be healthy, be beautiful, have fun, go places, see things, march up and get a diploma, dance, play ball, travel, etc. If "have sex" stays off your "to-do" list, you will probably get to do all these great things. How selfish can you get? Good, get that way!

Fact or Fiction–

People used to believe that the hymen was proof that a girl was a virgin. Now we know that the hymen always had an opening, which is often stretched open even further by regular physical activity.

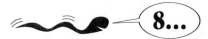

8...

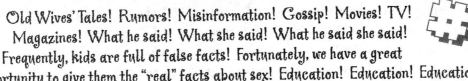

Flash!...Flash!...Flash!...Flash!... #4

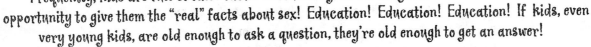

Old Wives' Tales! Rumors! Misinformation! Gossip! Movies! TV! Magazines! What he said! What she said! What he said she said! Frequently, kids are full of false facts! Fortunately, we have a great opportunity to give them the "real" facts about sex! Education! Education! Education! If kids, even very young kids, are old enough to ask a question, they're old enough to get an answer!

Q: Can I get pregnant from kissing?

A: No!

Q: Can I get pregnant from a swimming pool?

A: No!

Q: Can I get pregnant with my clothes on?

A: Yes!

Q: Can I get pregnant if I'm not married?

A: Yes!

Q: Can I get pregnant standing up?

A: Yes!

Q: Can I get pregnant during my period?

A: Yes!

Q: Can I get pregnant the first time I have sex?

A: Yes!

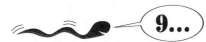

9...

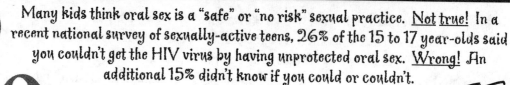
Many kids think oral sex is a "safe" or "no risk" sexual practice. <u>Not true!</u> In a recent national survey of sexually-active teens, 26% of the 15 to 17 year-olds said you couldn't get the HIV virus by having unprotected oral sex. <u>Wrong!</u> An additional 15% didn't know if you could or couldn't.

Q: What is "oral sex"?

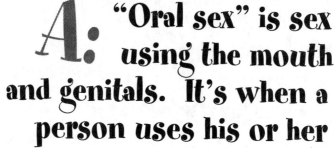

A: "Oral sex" is sex using the mouth and genitals. It's when a person uses his or her mouth or tongue to suck or lick a penis, a vagina, or an anus.

FACT!

Scientists <u>have</u> documented the transmission of other STDs, including herpes, syphilis, gonorrhea, and genital warts (HPV), intestinal parasites, and hepatitis during oral sex with an infected partner.

Q: Is "oral sex" really sex?

A: YES! Oral sex is frequently practiced by sexually-active couples, including adolescents. Today, more and more kids engage in oral sex thinking that they're not really "having sex"—but they are!

NOT!
Oral sex is not a safe "loophole" for teens who want to remain virgins.

Oral sex ≠ abstinence!
Oral sex ≠ safe sex!

AIDS can be transmitted through oral sex! Although the risk is less than during vaginal or anal sex, the HIV virus can be transmitted through oral sex!

FACT!

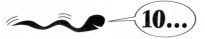 10...

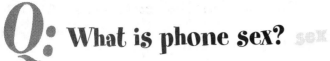

Flash!...Flash!...Flash!...Flash!...

Kids are bombarded daily with mounds of mind-boggling, state-of-the-art, hi-tech, techno-buddy-type info. On top of the heap is SEX, SEX, SEX! And every way imaginable to access it. Kids may understand how to get to the techno-buddy info better than their parents.

#6

Q: What is phone sex?

sex sex sex

A: Phone sex = sex over the telephone. There are numbers to call where a person will talk sexy to the caller. Some people masturbate while they listen. These calls cost money and are usually automatically charged to phone bills or credit cards—so, yes, Mom and Dad <u>will</u> find out!

Key Word

Pornography—writings or pictures designed to arouse sexual desire. "Porno" or "porn" for short!

Q: What is cybersex?

A: Cybersex = sex over the Internet. Recent U.S. government reports indicate one in five kids, aged 10 to 17, who regularly use the "Net" has been approached by a stranger wanting "cybersex." Nearly half of the advances were made by strangers believed to be 18 years old or younger. One quarter of the requests were believed to be made by young adults (18 to 25). More than two-thirds of the solicitations occurred while kids were using their computers at home.

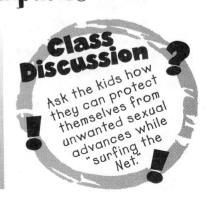

"Net" Fact:
The majoritiy of male Internet cybersex users studied visit sexual sites looking for pornography. Females usually visit "chat rooms" for sexy talk.

HOOKED ON PORN!
Hooked on porn! A recent study estimates that as many as 200,000 Internet users are "cybersex compulsives." That means they're hooked on pornographic sites or x-rated chat rooms. This sexual epidemic is just beginning to be uncovered.

Class Discussion
Ask the kids how they can protect themselves from unwanted sexual advances while "surfing the Net."

11...

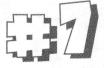

Hopefully you will find the tide changing and many kids not having sex as young, due to education—just as we have seen with drugs and smoking. You can remind kids of what happened with drugs and smoking—and how it was too late to help some kids. Sex will be the same way one day soon, and they don't want to wake up and find themselves a statistic they didn't have to be.

Q: What is casual sex?
(One girl guessed this meant having sex while wearing cut-off jeans and flip-flops!)

SLANG ALERT!
Friends with benefits = casual sex

A: Having sex with a person without planning or thinking about the consequences (what will happen), outside the bounds of a long-term relationship.

AIDS has put a real damper on casual sex. But that isn't so bad. All the reasons that casual sex wasn't a great idea in high school don't really change when you get older. You still don't want to accidentally get someone pregnant. You sure don't want to get a sex disease. So, you tend to have sex with someone you really care about and know. That's a lot more satisfying than a steamy, quick encounter with a girl at her house after school while you watch in a panic over your shoulder to be sure no parent is coming in the door!

SLANG ALERT!
Booty call = an invitation for casual sex

Q: Is any sex really safe?

A: Reality is that there are only <u>two ways</u> to have safe sex:

- **Not have sex at all**
- **Have sex <u>only</u> with the same partner over a very long period of time; a partner who has had sex <u>only</u> with you, and continues to have sex <u>only</u> with you**

It's a Must!

Kids need to understand that if they do have sex, they MUST use a condom and spermicides each and every time (even if the girl is on birth control pills) to protect against pregnancy and disease. They must understand that this is not the same as "safe" sex, it is only "safer sex" with precautions taken—precautions which are not always 100% safe and effective!

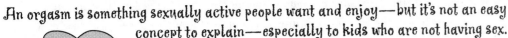

#8

An orgasm is something sexually active people want and enjoy—but it's not an easy concept to explain—especially to kids who are not having sex.

Q: What is an orgasm?

A: A very good and special feeling in your genitals that comes at the height of your sexual excitement. For a boy, this is when you ejaculate. For a girl, it's a throbbing shiver in the area of the clitoris or vagina. It lasts a short time, then you feel very relaxed. It's one of the things people enjoy most about sex. It feels good and it's nice to help your partner have this good feeling. You don't have to have sex with someone to have an orgasm. You may have one just thinking about sex, or while masturbating, or when you have sexual contact (but not necessarily intercourse) with another person.

Anatomy Fact

Within the folds of a girl's vulva, where the lips of flesh come to a point in the upper part of the pubic area, is the clitoris. This is a small, sensitive bump that feels so good when girls have an orgasm.

SLANG ALERT!

Come = semen or an orgasm

THEY USE WHAT?

Some people use *vibrators*, which are small devices held against the genitals to cause an orgasm. You might have felt the same sensation on a bouncing school bus.

13...

#9

Kids are involved with sex at a younger age. By age 19, 8 out of 10 boys and 7 out of 10 girls in the United States have had sexual intercourse. Two out of three say they don't use any regular birth control.

Q: What is birth control?

A: Planning the right time to get pregnant and have a baby. This is usually done by using contraceptives. Some types of contraceptives are: condoms; spermicide foam, cream, or jelly; birth control pills; IUD; and the diaphragm. Condoms, along with spermicides, are also used to try and prevent the spread of sexually transmitted diseases. Contraceptive sponges are currently off the market, but plans to reintroduce them are underway.

SLANG ALERT!
Rubber = condom

Contraceptives must be used the right way at the right time if you want them to work. People who do not believe in using artificial forms of birth control like those just listed, may try to avoid pregnancy by the rhythm method, or not having sex on the days when a female is most likely to get pregnant. No form of birth control is 100% guaranteed. This is why the best birth control for kids is to not have sex. Abortion should not be considered as a form of birth control. If a person is positive they never want to have children, they can have permanent birth control by being sterilized. This is a vasectomy for a male and tubal ligation (having the fallopian tubes tied) for a female.

There is so much in schools and on the news about kids and sex and kids and contraception and kids and pregnancy, that you may begin to feel like you don't have any choice except to figure out which form of contraception you are going to use, get it, and start having sex. NOT TRUE!

What the newspapers and adults often fail to say is that A LOT OF KIDS DON'T HAVE SEX until after high school, college, or they are married. Not having sex is a good choice—it just doesn't make many headlines. In fact, for many kids, it is the most common, logical, popular choice. If this is what you choose, you are very normal (and awfully smart!). No matter how the soap operas and movies and songs make it sound—no one "has" to have sex—even if you're in love!

Historical Facts! Historical Facts! Historical Facts!

For centuries there have been forms of coverings for the penis. Around 1350 BC, Egyptian men wore decorative covers over their penises. In 1564 these were made of cloth. Later, these protective covers were made from animal intestines. In the 18th century, they were first called condoms. People have also been very creative about contraceptives. Even 5000 years ago, women used a half of a lemon as a diaphragm.

14...

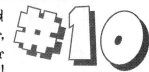

A baby pops out of its mother's belly button, right? <u>Wrong!</u> A baby's not delivered by the stork either. And it's not found in the cabbage patch! Kids need clear, candid communication. The information kids get from their friends can be <u>really wrong</u> and television can be <u>really dumb</u>!!

#10

Q: How do babies get out?

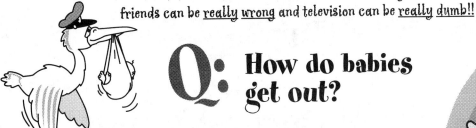

A: After a female becomes pregnant, the baby grows in the mother's uterus. Approximately nine months later, the baby travels down through the birth canal and is delivered through the vagina. This is called a natural delivery.

A baby can also be born by Caesarean section, which is when an opening is cut in the mother's abdomen and uterus to get the baby out.

Tell kids male seahorses have the babies!

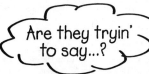

Are they tryin' to say...?

IT COULD HAPPEN!!!!

Biologists see no reason why an embryo fertilized in a lab cannot be implanted in a man's abdomen, which would later be delivered by a Cesarean section. (If you think I'm trying to say a man could have a baby—that's right. But there haven't been any volunteers yet—except in the movies!)

One boy thought a C-section was where the best basketball seats were!

15...

#11

Girls usually mature at an earlier age than boys. Let them know that what's happening to their bodies is normal. It happens to *all* girls, and it happens to *all* girls at *different* ages.

Q: What is puberty? What's happening to my body (for girls)?

A: One day, when you're around 9 or 10, the pituitary gland at the base of your brain says, "Yikes! It's time for this girl to grow up!" So it sends word to your body and slowly but surely, it yawns and stretches and gets down to the business of transforming a girl into a woman.

For a girl, maturing sexually includes the following. (While some may happen sooner or later, faster or slower, in sudden spurts or slowpokey, they eventually all happen in pretty much this order of events:)

1. The endocrine glands (pituitary, thyroid, parathyroids, and adrenals) send out chemicals called hormones into that highway in your body: Bloodstream One! This has been happening since you were born (*didn't hurt a bit, did it?!*), but now the hormones speed around faster and faster. Here's what the extra hormone activity causes:

● The dark circles around your nipples puff up. Next, the entire breast grows. One may grow faster than the other. They may ache. White, milky stuff may leak out. But it's all just part of the growing caused by those busy hormones.

It takes about three years for your breasts to do their growing up, so don't waste time being impatient or trying to help them along. (*Those "magic" creams don't work anyway.*) While growing girls worry if their breasts are too big or small, most women are very happy with the final results.

The female breast is a beautiful thing. If they weren't such an "up front" part of your body, they probably wouldn't receive all this attention. (*I mean, when's the last time you checked the size of the back of your knees?*) So, get your mom or a friend or a store clerk to help you pick out a pretty bra and enjoy your new-grown beauty!

➡ **Turn the page for more about puberty for girls.**

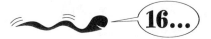

16...

What is Puberty–for Girls? (concluded)

● Hair begins to grow under your arms. The hair on your legs may get darker and stiffer. And hair begins to grow in the pubic area. In some countries, it's common for women to let the hair under the arms and on the legs grow naturally. In others, women usually shave their underarm and leg hair. I'm sure you and your mom can agree when the best time to start this practice will be.

Some girls may feel they're "growing a moustache," but this is just a little additional hair over your upper lip. If you have light hair, you may never notice it. If you have darker hair, it's easier to see. If it makes you uncomfortable or embarrassed, it can be simply *(but carefully!)* shaved off, or a dermatologist (skin doctor) can explain other remedies.

In fact, it's only because others can see (or you *think* they've noticed) that you pay so much attention to these outward changes. But really and truly, far more important things are happening!

2. Your reproductive organs, which are what make you able to have a baby, are also growing and changing.

The ovaries hold the eggs needed to create a baby. They begin to produce female hormones. These estrogens cause the reproductive organs to grow: the ovaries; the Fallopian tubes (that the eggs travel through to . . .); the uterus (where an egg may grow into a baby); and the vagina, which is the opening between your legs that leads to these reproductive organs.

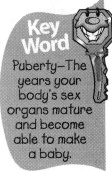

Key Word

Puberty–The years your body's sex organs mature and become able to make a baby.

3. Outside your vagina, the external genitals also change. In addition to hair growth, the vulva, which is the folds of skin and flesh around the opening of the vagina, begins to mature.

Just so we can get this straight: Yep, a girl has three outside openings between her legs:

• The urethra, which she urinates from.

• The anal opening, which her bowels move from.

• The vagina, which is used during sexual intercourse and is also the path a baby takes out of the mother's body when it's being born. This is also the opening she has her period from.

No, things don't all get mixed up or confused just because they are close together. I mean your eyes and nose are real close, but you don't "blow" your eye when you have a cold—even though you might "look down your nose" at someone?!

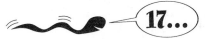 17...

#12

Let kids know that what's happening to their bodies is normal. It happens to everybody, and there is not any set age the body goes through it.

Q: What is puberty? What's happening to my body (for boys)?

A: The time when your body is physically able to become a father is called puberty. From the start of puberty to the time your body has reached complete physical maturity is called adolescence. During these years your body's sex organs mature and develop becoming able to make a baby. A boy's reproductive system begins to create sperm.

Maybe it seems strange that something as important as having a baby is so easy. You don't need lessons or a license. While it may take most of your teenage years to get your full height or grow a beard—one of the earliest things that happens to you during puberty is that you are able to make a baby.

You're smart enough to know that just because your body is suddenly capable of fathering a child, and just because you discover you have a dramatic new interest in girls and sex stuff—that emotionally you may not be ready for all this!

Relax, no one expects you to be. Adults—parents and teachers and older brothers and sisters and friends—are well-aware of the emotional changes that go along with growing up. After all, they've been through all this themselves.

There's no automatic set time boys begin to become men. A boy can reach puberty as young as age 10. Most boys reach puberty when they're about 13 or 14.

➡ Turn the page for more about puberty for boys.

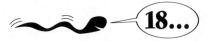 **18...**

What is Puberty–for Boys? (continued)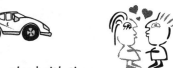

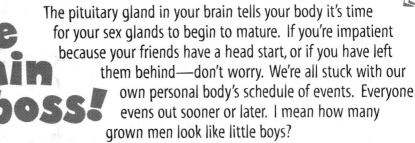

The pituitary gland in your brain tells your body it's time for your sex glands to begin to mature. If you're impatient because your friends have a head start, or if you have left them behind—don't worry. We're all stuck with our own personal body's schedule of events. Everyone evens out sooner or later. I mean how many grown men look like little boys?

Because of those active glands, you may perspire or sweat more than you used to. Normal.

You grow hair in the pubic area around your genitals. Hair grows under your arms, on your arms and legs, and possibly on your chest. At some point, you'll begin to grow hair on your face. The amount of hair and when a boy begins to grow it vary from boy to boy. Don't worry about it—about the time you finally get that hair on your face you may have longed for so bad, you may discover that shaving every day—if that is the custom where you live—may be more of a chore than a thrill!

Your voice loses its boyish sound and grows deeper. Your voice may sometimes "crack"—or start out on a word in a deep tone, then sort of squeak out the ending, or vice versa. This is normal, and pretty soon, your vocal chords will get used to their new sound and you won't have this problem anymore, so don't croak!

Acne. Zits. Pimples. Blackheads. Boys and girls often have problems with acne on their face and neck. Some kids have more trouble than others. These aggravating skin problems are caused by the changes in your body, so this should be a temporary problem. Everything that helps your body—good food, keeping clean, enough sleep—helps your skin. Your doctor or drug store pharmacist can suggest medication that might help your acne if it does not clear up.

Your entire body will begin to be shaped more like a man's and less like a boy's. Your shoulders grow broader. The muscles in your arms and legs develop more fully. Some soft and flabby "baby fat" you may put on while you are growing and changing disappears.

You usually don't get as tall as you're going to until age 18 or 19—so give yourself time! Also, all this new growth may make you seem clumsier for a while, but pretty soon, you'll be used to (and proud of!) your handsome new body.

The most important thing happening to you is probably the thing you're least aware of. Your testicles are starting to produce spermatozoa—sperm for short. The testicles also produce male hormones called androgens. The androgen called testosterone causes these physical changes in your body:
• Your testicles grow to about an inch around. The testicles are inside the scrotum, which is the sac of skin that hangs between your legs. It's normal for one sac to hang lower than the other. The testicles hang outside your body because sperm can't be produced inside—it's too warm.
• Your penis grows. It's outside the body because it's designed to be put inside the female vagina to deposit the sperm that will fertilize the egg that creates a new life.

 Turn the page for more about puberty for boys.

 19...

What is Puberty—for Boys? (concluded)

The sperm produced in the testicles moves on to a storage area called the epididymis. From there, the sperm enters the vas deferens which loops up and backward inside the body to join up with a seminal vesicle and the prostate.

In order to survive, the sperm cells mix with a milky, white fluid—semen. The semen carrying the sperm leaves the body like this:

• First, the penis gets stiff and hard. This is an erection. Blood flows into the spongy tissue of the penis. Sometimes, it gets stiff because you're sexually excited—thinking about girls, or reading a magazine or watching a movie that shows love scenes or "mushy stuff."

• A man's penis becomes erect so it can enter a woman's vagina to deposit sperm. When an erection occurs when you don't want it to or when it may be embarrassing, then you feel pretty miserable. But erections are as common and normal as can be.

• Once the penis is erect, another muscle contraction causes the semen to shoot out the end of your penis. This is an ejaculation. This is when a male has an orgasm. Sometimes the erection goes away and the semen is not ejaculated from the body. That's OK. The semen just stays in the body until later.

Even though the semen comes out the urethra, which is the same tube that urine comes out of when you go to the bathroom—urine and semen never pass through the tube at the same time.

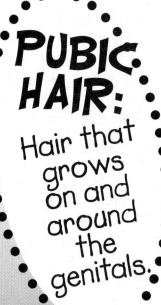

Sometimes boys worry about the size of their penis.

Penis size varies from man to man. There are a lot of myths about penis size that are not the least bit true. Here are a few of the things you should NOT believe:

• *The larger the penis, the more of a "man" you are.* Penis size has absolutely nothing to do with being "macho," becoming a father, or your ability to perform well sexually.

• *You can guess the size of a man's penis from the size of his hands or feet.* Not any more than I can guess the size of your ear by looking at your big toe!

• *Women prefer to have sexual intercourse with a man with a large penis rather than a small one.* Penis size is probably the last thing on any woman's list of "wants" as far as sex is concerned.

What's Up?

SOMETIMES THE PENIS GETS ERECT FOR NO APPARENT REASON. YOU MAY JUST BE MINDING YOUR OWN BUSINESS—RIDING YOUR BIKE OR TAKING A SHOWER. YOU MIGHT NOT PAY AS MUCH ATTENTION TO YOUR PENIS, OTHER THAN TO GO TO THE BATHROOM, IF IT DIDN'T BEGIN TO HAVE A MIND OF ITS OWN!

PUBIC HAIR: Hair that grows on and around the genitals.

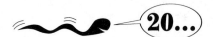

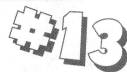

Although boys have questions about sex, we often ignore them. We think they already know the answers or will find out from their friends—not true! They need help understanding the sexual changes their bodies are going through, too.

#13

Q: What are wet dreams?

Sperm produced in the testicles moves on to a storage area called the epididymis. From there, the sperm enters the vas deferens which loops up and backward inside the body to join up with a seminal vesicle and the prostate. In order to survive, the sperm cells mix with a milky, white fluid—semen. When the semen carrying the sperm leaves the body, it does it like this:

First, the penis gets stiff and hard. This is an erection. Blood flows into the spongy tissue of the penis making the penis erect.

● Sometimes, it gets stiff for no apparent reason.
● Sometimes it gets hard because you're sexually excited—thinking about girls, or reading a magazine or watching a movie that shows love scenes or other "mushy stuff."
● A man's penis also becomes erect so it can enter a woman's vagina to deposit sperm.

Once the penis is erect, another muscle contraction causes the semen to shoot out the end of your penis. This is an ejaculation. This is when a male has an orgasm.

A: Sometimes you can have an erection and ejaculation at night while you are sleeping.

And Never The Twain Shall Meet:
Even though the semen comes out the urethra, which is the same tube that urine comes out of when you go to the bathroom—urine and semen never pass through the tube at the same time.

This is very normal. It's called a seminal emission (which sounds more like something related to your car, doesn't it?)–but you've probably heard it called a *wet dream*. This is the body's way of getting rid of semen it no longer has room to store. Sometimes you may wake up in the middle of a wet dream; other times you may sleep right through it.

Holding pattern:
Sometimes an erection goes away and the semen is not ejaculated from the body. That's OK. The semen just stays in the body until later.

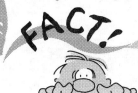

FACT!

Fact or Fiction–
Do all boys have wet dreams? No! Some boys never have wet dreams at all!

What's It Called?
What are "blue balls?" Just a colorful term to describe an ache in the groin or sex organs. This can happen when you have an erection for a long time without ejaculating. It'll go away once your sexual excitement is past. It might hurt, but it won't hurt you at all.

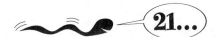

21...

#14

Let kids know masturbation is an option. Even adults use masturbation to relieve sexual frustration, so why should we discourage our kids from something that might provide a safety valve or a source of solace at various times during their lives?

Q: What is masturbation? Is it OK to do? Will it hurt you?

A: Masturbation is rubbing your own genitals. Boys and girls masturbate. Boys rub their penis making it erect. This usually causes an ejaculation. Girls rub their vulva, clitoris, and vagina. This may produce an orgasm. It won't make you go blind or cause hair to grow on your palms. Masturbation is not harmful or bad; in fact, it's a good alternative release for your sexual tensions and much safer than sex with another person. While you can overdo it—if that's all you do—if it helps relieve your sexual frustration and avoid sex and all the possible complications we've talked about, then try it. Most people masturbate at some time during their lives.

Why do you masturbate? It feels good. It's a natural way to learn about your body. From the time you're a baby, you're curious about how many of these you have, or what this hole is for. Even though you can read books, take a biology or sex-ed class, or "play doctor" with a friend—it's not the same as exploring your own body to see what's where and how it looks and feels. Don't be shy—get a mirror and look around!

Turn the page for more about masturbation. ➡

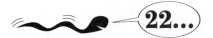

22...

What is Masturbation? (concluded)

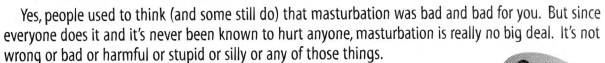

Yes, people used to think (and some still do) that masturbation was bad and bad for you. But since everyone does it and it's never been known to hurt anyone, masturbation is really no big deal. It's not wrong or bad or harmful or stupid or silly or any of those things.

This personal exploration of your body and how it responds is good preparation for the time when you'll let another person touch the sexual parts of your body. It not only makes you look forward to that time, it also makes you realize what a special time that will be, and not something that you'd want to share until the right time for you.

SLANG ALERT!
Spanking the monkey = Masturbation for guys

Do adults masturbate? Yes.

SLANG ALERT!
Stirring the soup = Masturbation for girls

Why? There's always more to learn about your body. Most people enjoy the sexual satisfaction masturbation can bring. While most adults probably prefer sharing their bodies with someone else, there are times in anyone's life when this is not possible or not a good idea.

When? Well, especially when you're too young to have sexual relations with another person. Our sex urges are very strong. Our minds know that sexual intercourse can bring pregnancy. And most kids know that a baby is something adults should have—not kids! So, masturbation is a way for us to satisfy some of our sexual needs without the risks that can accompany having sex with another person.

What kind of risks? Getting pregnant or getting a girl pregnant is the main problem. It's not a problem if you're married and settled and ready to have a family. But if you're still in school, perhaps planning on college or a job—the last thing you probably need is a baby!

As an adult you may masturbate for similar reasons. Maybe you don't want or have a steady girlfriend or boyfriend. Perhaps your husband or wife doesn't feel up to sex. You and your sex partner may be separated.

None of these things mean you lose your interest in sex. But as you can see, many times masturbation may be the most logical, easiest, safest, and satisfactory outlet for your sex needs.

Sum it Up!

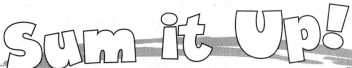

People used to think that masturbation was a bad habit. Now we know that it is just one way kids explore how their bodies feel and act. Kids may masturbate to help get rid of the strong sex urges they have (instead of having sex). Some girls and boys even masturbate one another instead of "having sex." Most people masturbate at some time during their lives.

23...

#15

About 80% of the world's population does not practice circumcision, including most residents of continental Europe and Asia (except Muslims), and most residents of the Western Hemisphere south of the United States.

Q: What does it mean to be circumcised?

A: <u>Circumcision</u> is the removal of the skin that covers the tip of the penis. If a penis is uncircumcised, there is a loose skin called the foreskin or prepuce that covers the <u>glans</u> or the tip of the penis. The word <u>circumcise</u> means to cut around. A surgeon removes the foreskin by cutting around the penis where the foreskin is attached.

All boys are born with a foreskin which covers the tip of the penis. Sometimes this skin is removed or circumcised soon after birth. Parents might decide to have a doctor remove this skin a day or two after a baby is born.

Traditionally, doctors in the U.S. have said that all baby boys should be circumcised. Some doctors used to say a lot of crazy things about circumcision. They thought it might prevent alcoholism, epilepsy, hernia, and lunacy—they were wrong. There is really only one medical benefit from circumcision; it makes the glans easier to clean, preventing infections.

Sometimes a substance called *smegma*—a product of glands located under the foreskin—can build up if it is not cleaned properly. Some doctors believe that smegma can cause cancer of the penis and the prostate, but there is no scientific evidence to prove this. In women, smegma can build up under the foreskin of the clitoris and it causes no harm.

There is nothing wrong with having an uncircumcised penis. But, research shows that uncircumcised males *are* more prone to infections of the urinary tract. Other doctors argue that properly cleaning the penis can prevent this.

For many religions the practice of circumcision is a *rite*—a ceremonial rule—practiced by that religion.

Turn the page for more about circumcision.

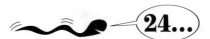

Male circumcision? (concluded)

Ancient artifacts discovered in Egypt show that circumcision has been practiced for thousands of years.

- Jewish males are circumcised at a special ceremony called a *bris milah* or bris for short. The ceremony is performed by someone qualified by Jewish law called a *mohel*.

- A Roman Catholic festival called Circumcision is celebrated on January 1, commemorating the circumcision of Jesus.

- Muslim boys are circumcised anywhere between the age of infancy to fourteen years old.

- Other groups including some Africans, Mayans, Aztecs, and Fiji Islanders also include circumcision as a rite of passage either when the boy is an infant or as late as puberty.

Female circumcision

You may think circumcision is something that only happens to boys, and most of the time that's true. In a few places in Africa and the Middle East, some people practice female circumcisions. When a circumcision is performed on a girl, some or all of the clitoris may be removed along with some of the labia. In a few cases, the operation is done to remove extreme cancer. But, usually this operation is not done for any medical reasons.

According to a recent United Nations report, fewer and fewer female circumcisions are being performed in Africa because many African women are against it.

No Medical Reason...

exists for female circumcision. In fact, the procedure may be done without anesthesia under unclean conditions. It's performed to remove the orgasmic parts of a girl's body as a social custom to keep her faithful to her eventual husband. Female circumcision leaves girls mutilated and often in pain!

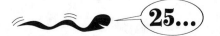

25...

#16

The media including television, newspapers, movies, and the Internet force adults to teach kids about stuff like this!

viagra-a

Q: **What is Viagra? What is a penile implant?**

A: **Wow, that's not one question, that's two! But, they are related. Viagra is a prescription drug that some men take to help them get an erection. Penile implants are medical devices men use to get an erection. See how they're related?**

When men get older, they may have trouble getting an erection once in a while. This is normal and may affect young men as well as older men. If a man has trouble getting an erection all of the time, there's something wrong. When a man cannot get an erection, it is called *impotence*. This might be caused by a disease, prescription medication, smoking, or alcoholism.

One way of treating impotence is by taking Viagra. The drug comes in pill form. Taking the drug will not automatically give a man an erection. The drug does increase blood flow to the penis so that when he is sexually aroused he can have an erection. There are other drugs for the treatment of impotence that are taken by injecting them into the penis.

IMPOTENCE

Drugs are not the only way to treat impotence. There are penis implants so that a man who could not have an erection—can, and therefore, happily continue his sex life. Will bionic genitals be next? There are different types of penile implants. Artificial rods can be surgically implanted into the penis. The penis is then always erect but can be bent close to the body to hide it. Another kind of penile implant is inflatable tubes. The tubes are placed in the penis along with a tiny pump. The pump is used to inflate the tubes making the penis erect.

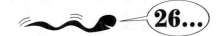

In spite of advances in sex education and contraceptive technology, nearly half of all pregnancies in the U.S. are not intended. Although U.S. abortion rates are down, current statistics from the CDC report 1,184,758 legal abortions are performed annually. That's 3,245 babies aborted every day! Twenty percent of those abortions were performed on women aged 19 and below.

#17

Q: What is an abortion?

A: Stopping a pregnancy on purpose before a baby is born. This is usually done during the first three months after you get pregnant. The only safe abortions are those done by a doctor. The doctor destroys the baby that is in the uterus. Many people believe that this is killing a baby. Many people feel the girl should be able to choose whether or not she wants to continue her pregnancy. Most people agree that an abortion is the best thing to do if a girl's life is in danger or if she has been raped. Most people also agree that abortion is definitely not a form of birth control.

While some girls may not worry if they get pregnant—because they can get an abortion—this is not a good idea. Why? Because you may feel as confused as adults do about the right of the baby to live versus the right of the mother to stop the pregnancy. The father may feel he should have the right to make a decision. In other words, getting pregnant is EASY; the decisions and choices you face afterwards can be very hard—on your body and your mind. Something new under the "after-the-fact" sun is the so-called Morning After Pill. Legal in some countries, it is a pill a girl takes after she has had sex. It may prevent, or end, a conception, if it occurs.

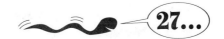

27...

#18

Child abuse is one of the saddest things we know about. It really seems unbelievable that anyone could hurt a child of any age. But we know that sexual abuse of children is a fact of life. Sexual abuse was one of those subjects people used to just not talk about. But now everyone knows that such problems exist.

Q: What is rape?

A: Rape is when someone forces you to have sex with them. It is against the law for anyone to do this.

We usually think of rape as being something very violent. And rape is an act of violence—it is the most frequently committed violent crime in the United States! But, that does not necessarily mean that it is a dark night and someone you don't know forces you into their car and makes you have sex with them. The majority of rapes are committed by someone the victim knows—*not* by a stranger!

No matter how innocent things may start out: a date; kissing in the back seat of the car; or messing around at home while your parents are at work—no one has the right to force you to have sex with them. If they do, they are guilty of a crime.

They may have a hard time understanding this. *"I thought they wanted to." "They didn't say no." "You can't tease someone, then change your mind."* But thinking someone wants to have sex is *not* the same thing as them agreeing to have sex. Not saying no is *not* the same thing as saying yes.

• •

You <u>can</u> change your mind. That goes for boys, as well as girls. Boys should understand that having sex with a minor (underage girl) is a crime!

• •

NO! means NO!

Rape is against the law!!!

Rape is not something that is your fault or that you made happen. Understand how easy and fast it can happen in your own home or on a date. Imagine yourself in such situations and plan ahead how you would respond. Then try to avoid any situation that could make you a target for such abuse.

Classroom Activity

Pair the kids up and let them practice saying "NO!!!" to each other.

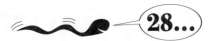

A lot of kids don't think they can get any of the following diseases if they keep themselves clean, don't have sex very often, or have one, steady sex partner. Sorry, but this is just not true! Not at all!

#19

Q: What are STDs?

A: Sexually transmitted diseases are exactly that: diseases that are passed from one person to another during sex.

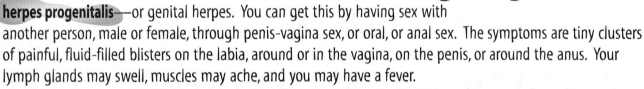

STD High-Risk
STD High-Risk

You mean it's not motor oil?

Sexually Transmitted Diseases can infect anyone. You can get infected the first—and only—time you have sex. You can be infected by the nicest, cleanest kid you know. What are these diseases?

herpes progenitalis—or genital herpes. You can get this by having sex with another person, male or female, through penis-vagina sex, or oral, or anal sex. The symptoms are tiny clusters of painful, fluid-filled blisters on the labia, around or in the vagina, on the penis, or around the anus. Your lymph glands may swell, muscles may ache, and you may have a fever.

Symptoms show up 2-20 days after you're infected and usually diminish or disappear after a few weeks. BUT, the virus is still in your body. While symptoms may never reappear, it's FAR MORE COMMON that they do. You don't have to have sex again to trigger an attack. It can come when you are tired, sick, or under stress—such as during exams. Before an attack and while you have sores, you can give the disease to someone else if you have sex with them. Although some drugs help relieve the symptoms, there's no cure for herpes at this time.

chlamydia—A woman may have vaginal irritation or no symptoms at all. A man will have a discharge from the penis and may have painful urination. Antibiotics are used to treat the disease. Chlamydia is the most common bacterial STD in the U.S. If left untreated, chlamydia can lead to infertility. Recent studies indicate that chlamydia can increase the risk of cervical cancer in women who are also infected with human papilloma virus (HPV).

gonorrhea—Bacteria live in the warm, wet places of the penis, cervix, throat, or rectum, and are transmitted through sexual contact.

Turn the page for more about STDs.

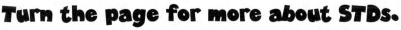

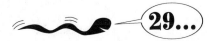
29...

STDs (continued)

Males usually have symptoms 2-9 days after they are exposed to the disease. They may have painful urination and an uncomfortable, thick, yellowish discharge from the penis. If the throat or rectum is infected, they may have a sore throat, rectal pain and itching, and mucus in the bowel movements.

Women usually have NO symptoms until much later. By then, pelvic or lower abdominal pain can mean the undetected disease has developed into a more serious pelvic inflammatory disease. An untreated disease can cause sterility in women, problems with joints, and even in heart valves, in men and women. The disease is treated with antibiotic pills or penicillin shots.

Gonorrhea transmitted from the vagina to a baby's eyes during birth can make the child blind. Most hospitals put silver nitrate in newborn babies' eyes to prevent this.

syphilis—is usually spread by sexual contact, but you can also get it if an infected sex organ touches an open cut anywhere on your skin. Symptoms show up in three stages:

• First, 10-90 days after you are exposed, there might be a painless sore on the genitals, rectum, lips or mouth, that disappears in a week or two.

• A few weeks or even months later, you might discover a rash all over your body. Your joints may swell, and you may feel like you have the flu. These symptoms will go away too, but you will still have the disease, so you can see why it's important to have symptoms checked out immediately. If detected early, it can be cured.

• It may be years before the final stage of the disease appears. You may discover you have damage to the nervous system, brain and/or circulatory systems. This damage can lead to heart problems, insanity, paralysis, and possibly, death. A mother can give a baby syphilis. This can result in it being born dead or with deformed bones, blind, or a disfigured face.

human papilloma virus infection (HPV)—or genital warts, sounds like something that a frog trying to make love to a rock should get, but it's not. It is caused by a virus and transmitted during sex. About a month or so after you are exposed, you may find skin-colored, cauliflower-shaped bumps around your vagina, rectum, or penis. They may itch and feel irritated. You need to see a doctor fast. Why? Because they can spread fast and cover the entire genital area. A doctor will remove the warts—and you should only let a *doctor* do this. There are several ways to remove them: with medication; burn off with an electric needle; or freeze off with liquid nitrogen. HPV may cause cancer of the cervix or penis.

pubic lice—are six-legged parasites that live and lay eggs in pubic hair. If you have sex with someone who has pubic lice, these "crabs" will be happy to jump right over to you! You can also get them from bedding, clothes, towels, and toilet seats which have been infected.

You can tell you have crabs because you can see them and their eggs in your pubic hair. You'll also itch "where you can't scratch" something awful! You might see tiny spots of blood on your underwear that comes from places where the lice have burrowed under the skin. If you can see this on you—you can also see it on

Turn the page for more about STDs.

STDs (concluded)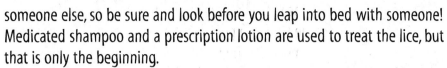

someone else, so be sure and look before you leap into bed with someone! Medicated shampoo and a prescription lotion are used to treat the lice, but that is only the beginning.

You must wash bedding, towels and clothes in very hot water to get rid of the lice and any eggs. Also, you can't have sex for at least a week. And, if you have sex again with the person you got them from (who maybe even got them from you?!) before they've been treated—you'll just get them all over again. Is all that itching and washing and misery worth it? NOT!

scabies—is caused by a mite. You can get it via sex, close skin-to-skin contact, or infected bedding, clothes and blankets. You'll know you have it from the awful itching—especially at night.

Where the mite burrows under the skin, you may see red spots or raised red or gray lines. This can happen on the genitals, buttocks, breasts, hands, or elbows. A prescription cream, more washing, and no sex will treat it.

tinea cruris—"jock itch" or "jock rot." You can get this fungus that gives you a scaly, itchy rash in the crotch from an unwashed athletic supporter or jock strap. *Girls*, you can get it from guys during skin-to-skin sexual contact! It is treated with medication you can buy at the drug store, but if it doesn't get better, you'll need a prescription from a doctor for something stronger. You also need to dry off good after a shower or swim, wear cotton underwear, and no tight jeans.

trichomoniasis—is something else you can get sexually or from towels, washcloths, or bathing suits. It's an infection of the vagina or man's urethra. A woman would have a frothy, yellow-green discharge that smells bad; painful, frequent urination; itching; a red, swollen vulva; and maybe severe lower abdominal pain. Men may only have a little pain in the penis. Both partners must take pills.

YOU CAN HELP AVOID GETTING A SEXUALLY TRANSMITTED DISEASE BY: USING GOOD HYGIENE, ESPECIALLY BEFORE AND AFTER SEX—AND INSISTING YOUR PARTNER DOES TOO; USING CONDOMS ALONG WITH SPERMICIDES; EXAMINING A SEX PARTNER'S GENITALS FOR SYMPTOMS; AND NOT HAVING SEX WITH ANYONE WHO HAS SYMPTOMS.

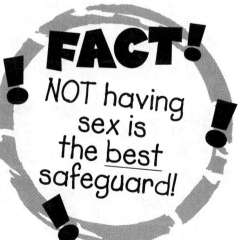

FACT! NOT having sex is the best safeguard!

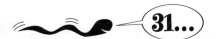

31...

For years now, kids have heard about AIDS, AIDS, AIDS. Like many adults, they assume that it only affects homosexuals, and that there is a cure. Neither is true!

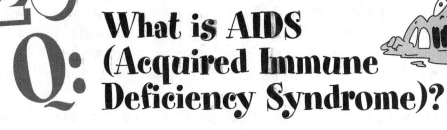

#20
Q: What is AIDS (Acquired Immune Deficiency Syndrome)?

A: AIDS is a disease that cripples the immune system. You can get it:

- By having sex with someone who has it. This can be a male or female.
- By using a needle for drugs that someone with AIDS has already used.
- Through infected blood.

You *can't* get AIDS just from being around someone who has it, even if you touch, hug or kiss them, or eat a sandwich they made, for example.

Discussion Question?
Ask the students if they know anyone who has AIDS? If yes, how does it make them feel?

How you can best avoid any risk of getting AIDS!

- By not having sex until you are old enough to choose one sex partner and stick with them (and they with you) for years and years. Yes, this is usually when you get married. The thing you want to avoid is having sex with many different partners. After all, you don't know who they have had sex with!
- By not using drugs at all, especially by needle injection.
- By staying informed about new information on this disease.

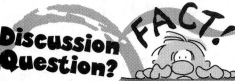

Discussion Question?
Ask the students if they think a cure will ever be found for AIDS?

FACT!
AIDS is carried and transmitted in blood, semen, and vaginal secretions. You can get AIDS anytime semen or vaginal secretions touch you if that person is infected with the virus. Since this most usually happens during sex, that is the main way the disease is transmitted.

There is no cure for AIDS at this time! However, there are medications that can help HIV (human immunodeficiency virus) and AIDS patients. If you have HIV or AIDS and get pregnant, your baby can be born infected with the virus.

Using condoms and spermicides will prevent AIDS, *right?* WRONG! These protective measures will only reduce the risk of getting AIDS!

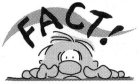
FACT!
AIDS leaves a person more likely to get many kinds of very infectious or contagious diseases that can kill them.

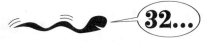
32...

Today, the world's oldest profession is employing some of the world's youngest employees! Children as young as 10 years old are being lured into the sex trade, exploited, and jailed while their adult pimps go free.

#21

Q: What is a prostitute?

A: Person who gets paid to have sex.

Q: What is a pimp?

A: Person who finds customers for a prostitute in return for a portion of the prostitute's earnings.

Kids are caught up in what once was the adult world of prostitution. Since the late 1970s, child prostitution has become a growing problem in the U.S. In 1974, the U.S. Congress passed the Juvenile Justice Delinquency Prevention Act which prevented police from arresting children for running away from home. This meant runaway kids had to find a way to support themselves. Selling their bodies for sex became a way of life. Prostitutes can be male or female. In most countries, it's illegal. Kids who run away from home and kids on drugs often turn to prostitution. Having sex with a lot of different partners can be very hazardous to your health.

Key Word
Exploit—take unfair advantage of

Fact! Prostitutes have a high risk of getting a STD because they have a lot of different sex partners. If you have sex with someone who is or has been a prostitute (whether you know it or not), you have increased your risk of getting AIDS. You never really know when someone has spent some time as a prostitute and therefore had sex with different people.

It's not so funny anymore!

While once some people thought it was fun or a joke or a treat to arrange for a young boy to have sex with a prostitute, this is obviously no longer a wise idea.

Help is on the way!

Pimps: Low-life, bottom-sucking, pond-scum

More and more Americans are becoming aware of this desperate problem and trying to help these kids who've turned to prostitution. Laws to make "pimping" a serious crime are being considered so that the pimps—not the children—will be punished!

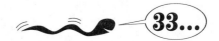 33...

#22

Your sexual preference is a part of you—the way you are and were meant to be. If a heterosexual and a homosexual made a list of all the ways they are alike (including "want to be loved, want to have a home, like ice cream"), they would find a very long list. If they list the ways they are different, "Like other guys/Prefer girls"—might be the only thing on that list!

Q: What does "gay" mean?

A: As some people mature, they realize they are sexually attracted to members of their own sex. They are <u>homosexuals</u>. <u>Homosexual</u> men, or gays, prefer to have sex only with other men. Homosexual men have sex either orally (one puts his penis in the other's mouth) or anally (putting the penis in the anus).

IF A BOY DOESN'T LIKE GIRLS, DOES THAT MEAN HE'S GAY?

No! Give puberty time to set in. When it does, some of the strong new emotions are exciting; others seem a real bother. I mean you were pretty good at thinking girls were a big pain in the neck...and now you're afraid you might actually be beginning to like them. *Yikes!*

SLANG ALERT!
Coming out of the closet = telling people about being homosexual

Key Word
Homophobia—hatred, intense disapproval, or fear of homosexuals and their culture. People are often frightened by things that are different or they don't understand!
Homosexuals are intentionally persecuted apparently only because they're gay! Sometimes, persecution leads to death!

Both Sides!
No matter your personal opinion on subjects of a sexual nature, it's only fair to give kids both sides of any sex story so they can better understand the complex issues involved!

34...

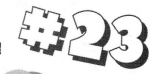

Ongoing debate: What causes a person to be a homosexual? Sexuality experts do not believe people choose to be or not to be. Research indicates it might be in our jeans—oops! genes, although nurturing may play a role in this still little-understood process.

#23

Q: What is a lesbian?

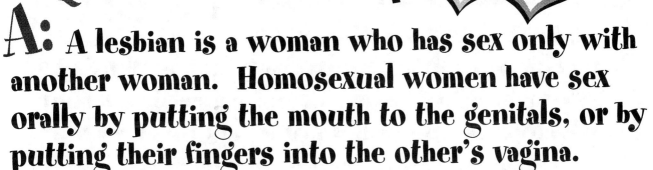

A: A lesbian is a woman who has sex only with another woman. Homosexual women have sex orally by putting the mouth to the genitals, or by putting their fingers into the other's vagina.

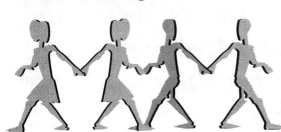

We're not talking about a girl having a crush on a female teacher. Many girls and boys try out at least one sexual activity with someone of their own sex. This doesn't mean they're "homosexual"—it's just another part of the early exploration of their sexuality.

#24 •

Q: What does bisexual mean?

A: A person who has sex with other people of the same sex, and with people of the opposite sex = males with males + males with females. Also = females with females + females with males.

Sometimes, a person discovers they are *transsexual*. Even though their body may have male or female sex organs, in their brain, they know they are really the opposite sex. Sometimes, they have surgery to alter their sex organs. *Transvestites* are people who like to dress in clothes of the opposite sex, usually men who like to dress like women.

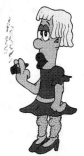

35...

The Big "C!" Terrifying—Yes! Always fatal—No! Early detection is the key to beating cancer—the key to making it just another regular-old little "c"!

#25

Q: What is breast cancer?

A: Cancer is a harmful or deadly growth (tumor) that happens when cells multiply uncontrollably in a person's body destroying healthy tissue. Breast cancer is a tumor that develops in one or both of a person's breasts.

Early detection through self-examination and checkups with a doctor is the key to fighting and surviving breast cancer!

FACT!

Men can get breast cancer, too. But, the number of men that get breast cancer is much smaller than the number of women that get it. In the U.S., about 400 men die each year from breast cancer.

More than 40,000 women in the U.S. die from breast cancer each year. With early detection and treatment, the five-year survival rate is about 95 percent. Today, there are about 2 million breast cancer survivors *living* in the U.S.

Do kids get breast cancer? No, cancer in women younger than 30 is very rare.

Q: What is testicular cancer?

A: Cancer that occurs in a man's testicles—the egg-shaped glands below the penis, in the scrotum. It's the most common form of cancer among men aged 15 to 35, BUT, it's one of the most treatable cancers when it's caught early! Regular checkups with your family doctor will detect any problems.

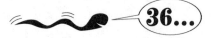

36...

Tips & Guidance for Parents and Teachers

Congratulations on your brave and courageous attempt to help kids struggling with questions about sex stuff. I know it is difficult to know if you should answer, how you should answer, and why you should answer. Here are a few tips to help guide you:

● If a child is old enough to ask a question, he or she is old enough to get an answer.

● Take time to ascertain just what the question is—it may not be about sex at all!

● Give an honest answer.

● Give an accurate answer.

● If you don't know, or need time to think about your response, say so and tell the child when you will get back with them with an answer.

● Keep your answer short! "I only wanted an answer," one kid said, "not an encyclopedia!" Kids will ask follow-up questions if they want to.

● Plan ahead! If it's on the nightly news, you may get a question the next morning—so think of how you might answer.

● Use real words: these give you communication building blocks so that you can get past the body parts, and the reproductive plumbing explanation, so you can get to the important stuff—relationships and responsibilities!

● Don't miss that fourth grade window of opportunity, when they're not shy about asking, are genuinely curious, and generally respond just like you want them to ("Yuck! Who wants to do that?!").

● Give both sides of an issue; don't preach; give scenarios and let kids draw their own conclusions, just like they'll have to in real life.

● Think kids have ulterior motives for asking provocative questions? Perhaps something is going on in their lives that needs special attention. Please don't ignore them—they need your help!

● Form sex ed partnerships with parents, fellow teachers, school and community resources, and others. Even pediatricians have come out opposed to the barrage of sexual images our youth see each day! Lots of sex with little talk of possible negative consequences! Let's all be on the same side—the smart sex side!

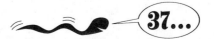

37...

Helpful Handouts for Healthy Kids!

SIX SMART SEX STEPS: For Virgins
If I find myself being tempted, teased, or threatened into sex, I WILL:

1. Do what I would want my younger brother or sister to do!

2. Do what I would **honestly** want my own kid to do!

3. Do what will make tomorrow **better**—not *worse!*

4. Do what I will be **very** happy/relieved/proud I did, in the morning, in a week, next month, *in nine months!*

5. Do what I/Me/My own **real** self really and truly wants to do and knows is *best* for me!

6. **Just say No! Don't do it! Chicken out!**

SIX SMART SEX STEPS: For the Sexually Active
If I think I might have sex, have sex one time, or have sex regularly, I WILL:

1. Prepare **AHEAD OF TIME** to protect myself against pregnancy and disease.

2. Ask my partner about their sexual history and decide if I'm hearing the **truth** or *not.*

3. **INSIST** a condom and spermicide are used, and be ready to provide both, or **STOP**.

4. Be **sure** my partner and I know how to contact one another in case either develops symptoms or tests positive for a sexually transmitted disease in the future.

5. Watch myself for *any* symptoms of disease since I'm aware this is a possibility as long as I am sexually active.

6. Have any symptom checked **immediately** since I know even if it "goes away," that *doesn't* mean the disease is gone.

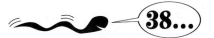

38...

My Lifetime of Sexuality Timeline

My Lifetime of Sexuality Timeline

Here are just some of the things that can be part of your sex life. To complete the timeline, have kids fill in the circles that best show when these events will occur throughout their lives.

	Have more sex	Be celibate	Have lots of sex	Practice birth control	Have children	Get married	Practice safe sex	Decide to abstain from sex until marriage	Go "out" (go steady)	Have lots of girlfriends/boyfriends	Get first kiss	Have first date	Go thru puberty	Be in puppy love	Wonder what sex is all about	See sexy stuff on tv	play doctor, see other kids naked	Ask where babies come from	Learn body part names
100 YEARS OLD	○	○	○	○	○	○	○	○	○	○	○	○	○	○	○	○	○	○	○
70-90s	○	○	○	○	○	○	○	○	○	○	○	○	○	○	○	○	○	○	○
50-60s	○	○	○	○	○	○	○	○	○	○	○	○	○	○	○	○	○	○	○
40s	○	○	○	○	○	○	○	○	○	○	○	○	○	○	○	○	○	○	○
30s	○	○	○	○	○	○	○	○	○	○	○	○	○	○	○	○	○	○	○
20-29	○	○	○	○	○	○	○	○	○	○	○	○	○	○	○	○	○	○	○
18-19	○	○	○	○	○	○	○	○	○	○	○	○	○	○	○	○	○	○	○
15-17	○	○	○	○	○	○	○	○	○	○	○	○	○	○	○	○	○	○	○
12-14	○	○	○	○	○	○	○	○	○	○	○	○	○	○	○	○	○	○	○
7-11	○	○	○	○	○	○	○	○	○	○	○	○	○	○	○	○	○	○	○
1-6	○	○	○	○	○	○	○	○	○	○	○	○	○	○	○	○	○	○	○
BIRTH	○	○	○	○	○	○	○	○	○	○	○	○	○	○	○	○	○	○	○

Signed: _____

Date and Age: _____

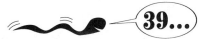

39...

"Scary Facts" Fact Sheet

HIV/AIDS/STDs

● In 1998, HIV was the fifth leading cause of death in the United States for men and women aged 25 to 44.

● Estimates now indicate that at least half of all new HIV infections in the U.S. affect men and women under age 25—the majority of whom are infected through sexual activity.

● In 1999, young people, aged 13 to 24, reported to be infected with AIDS in the U.S. totalled 29,629!

● An estimated 12 million STD cases other than HIV are diagnosed annually in the U.S. About two-thirds of these cases are young people under the age of 25!

Teen Prostitution

● Estimates on the number of child runaways indicate more than one million kids leave home each year. About one-third of these runaways become involved with pornography and/or prostitution.

● Today, International Relief Organizations estimate there are more than 300,000 children under the age of 16 working as prostitutes in the U.S.

Teen Pregnancy

● Since the early 1990s, teen pregnancy and births (girls aged 15-19) have been declining in the U.S. (that's good news!)—BUT—4 out of 10 girls still get pregnant at least once before they are 20 years old (that's NOT good news!). The U.S. still has the highest teen pregnancy and birth rate of any industrialized country in the world!

The U.S. Centers for Disease Control and Prevention's research has shown that early communication about sex between parents and kids is a critical step in helping our youth learn, adopt, and maintain life-saving, protective sexual behaviors. School-based programs are also a crucial element in reaching kids before sexual behaviors are established. The most effective programs focus on delaying sex and giving sexually-active kids information on how to protect themselves!

....

A poll asked:
"Do you and your parents discuss sex?"
49% of parents said "Yes!"
But only 23% of their kids agreed!

 40...

Silly and Strange but True Sex Stuff Trivia!

Want to get paid a real compliment? How would you like to overhear "Ms. Jones knows the coolest stuff about sex." The things that are TRUE about sex can be more surprising than anything you'll ever make up! Let's take a look at just a sampling of how wide a variety of sex exists:

● Sex between a male and a female isn't even necessary for reproduction in some species! *(Aren't we glad that doesn't include us!)*

● *Trichonymphas*—live in the intestines of termites and cockroaches and can turn into a male or female. The small male enters the larger female completely! Sometimes a male gets mixed up and climbs into another male. *("Oops! Excuse me!!")*

● Consider the sex life of an oyster. They spend all their time in "beds," but can't get together with the opposite sex because they are anchored in place. *(Talk about being "stuck" without a date!)*

● In the fall, the Samoan palolo worm becomes a sex machine and has the sea frothing in an orgy just before dawn on the first day of the last quarter of the October and November moons! *(Mark your calendar!)*

● Grunion "run" out of the water, up on the sand, swirl and writhe, and go back into the sea sexually satisfied—all in about 25 seconds!

● Scientists say if creatures live in large groups (mostly female), it's better to be a male, and vice versa. *(But, I think we could have figured that out for ourselves, don't you?)*

● The male wrasse fish has a harem of several females. If he dies, the largest, oldest female takes his place by becoming a male!

● The male seahorse has the babies in that family!

● A scorpion fly is long and thin. The male is so lazy, it finds it easier to get sex and food by pretending to be a female and attracting a male!

 41...

● The ruffed grouse "drums" up a sex partner by making a drumming noise. It's hard to tell girl drumming from boy drumming. If a male "drums" and another grouse shows up and punches him—he knows it's another male. If a grouse shows up and ignores him—it's a female. Sometimes they mistake the sound of a farm tractor for drumming and get friendly with the machine!

● Earthworms, or night crawlers, each have a male and a female sex organ—which fertilize each other!

● Sea cucumbers and sea hares form a long chain and reproduce, as many as 12 at a time— each one gives sperm to the next!

● When helix snails meet, they press a part of their foot against one another and feel each other all over with tentacles and lips. They each have a penis which they put into the other to exchange sperm.

● Consider the sex life of a slug (ugh?!) They hang from a tree branch and mate in mid-air, twist together, and insert club-shaped penises into each other. When they are done, they fall to the ground. *(I would, too, wouldn't you?!)*

● Aphids or plant lice produce live young which live inside the parent. These live young can produce live young which live inside them while they live inside, etc. *(Saves rent?)*

● Whiptail lizards are female and hatch only females! *Huh?*

● Giant Japanese male spider crabs have twin penises shaped like corkscrews!

● The sex life of a Chinese bamboo plant occurs only once around the world—every 120 years!

● In their dark sea home, anglerfish have a hard time finding one another. The female is large, the male tiny. When they do get together, the male becomes a parasite on the female. Since she gives him both food and sex, he can never let her go. *(I saw a soap opera like this once!)*

● Fireflies or lightning bugs are actually flirting with their lights!

● It's no wonder the male praying mantis prays—the female eats him alive from the head down during sex.

● The male toad must cling to the female toad's back for 3-26 days to mate. Sometimes the male is so eager to have sex that he climbs onto the back of a rock by mistake!

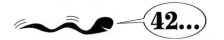 42...

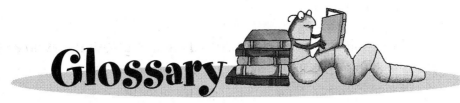

Glossary

Abortion: Stopping a pregnancy before a baby is born
Abstinence: Choosing not to do something
Adolescence: Pre-teen thru teen years
Adultery: Married people having sex with someone other than their spouses
AIDS: A disease you can get from having sex; it kills you
Anorexia: Dieting to the extent it makes you very sick
"Anteater": uncircumcised boy
Anus, anal: Opening your bowels move from
Baby: What kids who have sex often end up with
"Beaver": Female genitals
Birth control: Ways to try to prevent pregnancy
Bisexual: Person who has sex with the same and the opposite sex
"Booty Call": An invitation for casual sex
Brain: Your main sex organ
Breasts: Glands on a girl's chest; used to feed milk to a baby
Bulimia: Overeating and then vomiting to try to stay thin
Cancer: Harmful or deadly tumor that destroys healthy cells
Casual Sex: Having sex with a person without planning or thinking about the consequences (what will happen) outside the bounds of a long-term relationship
Celibacy: Deciding not to have sex
Cervix: Opening to the uterus
Chlamydia: A sexually transmitted disease
Circumcision: The removal of the foreskin of the penis
Clitoris: Small bump of flesh in the female genitals
"Come": Slang word for semen or an orgasm
"Coming out of the closet": telling people about being homosexual
Condom: A thin piece of rubber over the penis to contain sperm
Contraception: Ways to try to prevent pregnancy
"Crabs": Tiny bugs in pubic hair; lice
Cramps: Aches in the abdomen before a girl's period
Cunnilingus: To kiss, lick, or suck a woman's genitals. Slang = *"carpet munching"*
"Cybersex": Sex over the Internet
Dating: Going out with someone of the opposite sex for fun and friendship
Diaphragm: A rubber cup that fits over the cervix to keep sperm out
Douching: Squirting water into the vagina to clean it
Drugs: Chemicals that can kill you
Egg: In the female, it combines with a sperm to make a baby
Ejaculation: When semen squirts from the penis during a male orgasm
Erection: When the penis gets stiff and hard
Ethics: Generally agreed-upon rules people follow to have a better society in which to live and work
Father: What you become if you get a girl pregnant
Fellatio: To kiss, lick, or suck a penis. Slang = *"giving head"*
Fertile: To be able to get pregnant
Fertilization: When a sperm enters an egg and begins a baby
Foam: A contraceptive you squirt in the vagina before sex
Fornication: Sex between unmarried people
Friends: People who don't try to pressure you into having sex
"Friends with benefits": Casual sex
Fun: What you can have a lot more of a lot longer if you don't have sex!
Gay: A homosexual

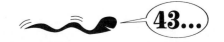 43...

Glossary (continued)

Genitals: The sex organs on the outside of your body
Gonorrhea: A contagious sex disease
"Helmet": circumcised boy
Herpes: A contagious sex disease
Heterosexual: A person who prefers sex with someone of the opposite sex
Homosexual: A person who prefers sex with someone of the same sex
Hormones: Chemicals that cause your body to change and grow
"Horny": Feeling like you want to have sex
Human papilloma virus infection (HPV): A contagious sex disease
Hymen: Thin piece of skin that partly covers the opening to the vagina
Immaturity: Acting childish—no matter what your age
Intercourse: The putting of the penis into the vagina
IUD: IntraUterine Device; used for contraception
Jock itch: Rash in the pubic area
Kinky sex: Unusual sex acts
Labia: Lips of flesh in the female pubic area
Lesbian: Female homosexual
"Louisville Slugger": Male's penis
Love: Intense affection and sexual attraction to another person
Marriage: Commitment to be sexually faithful to one another
Masochist: Person who gets sexual pleasure from pain
Masturbation: Rubbing your sex organs for sexual pleasure
Maturity: Acting grown up—no matter what your age
Menopause: When a woman quits having her periods
Monogamy: Only having sex with the same person all the time
Morals: Beliefs about right and wrong
Mother: What you will be if you get pregnant and have a baby
Nipples: Tip ends of the male or female breast
"No!" A very important word in your sexual vocabulary
Normal: What you are!
"Old Wives' Tales": Things people say about sex that aren't true
Oral sex: Sex using the mouth and the genitals
Orgasm: A good feeling that can happen during intercourse or masturbation
Orgy: A group of people having sex
"Outercourse": Necking and petting, but not ending with sexual intercourse
Ovaries: Where the eggs to make a baby come from
Ovulation: The release of one of these eggs
Parent: What you will automatically have in common with your mom or dad if you have a baby
Peer pressure: People your own age who try to get you to do things you both know you shouldn't so you can all get in trouble together
Penis: The male sex organ outside the body
Period: Time of month when a female menstruates
"Phone" sex: Sex over the telephone
Pill, The: Oral contraceptive taken to try to prevent pregnancy
Pimp: Person who finds customers for prostitutes for a portion of the money earned for having sex
PMS: Pre (before) Menstrual (period) Syndrome (symptoms)
Pornography: Pictures and writing designed to stimulate sexual desire
Pregnancy: The fertilization of the female's egg by a male's sperm and the nine months it takes for this to grow into a baby
Promiscuous: Having sex with different people
Prostitute: Person who gets paid to have sex
Puberty: The time of your sexual development
Pubic hair: Hair that grows on and around the genitals

44...

Glossary (concluded)

Rape: The forcing of someone to have sex when they do not agree to it

Reproduction: The creating of new life through sex and pregnancy

Responsibility: What you must take for your sex life

Rhythm: Trying to not get pregnant by not having sex on the days you think you might be most likely to get pregnant

Romance: What many people really want instead of sex

"Rubber": A slang name for a condom

Sadist: A person who enjoys sex that is painful

Safe Sex: No sex, or sex for a very long period of time *only* with someone who has had sex *only* with you and continues to have sex *only* with you

Sanitary napkin: Throw-away pads a girl wears during her period

Scabies: A disease that can be transmitted sexually

"Score": Slang term for getting someone to have sex with you

Scrotum: The sac of skin the male testicles are in

Selfish: Something good to be when it comes to sex

Semen: Sperm and other substances that come out when a boy ejaculates

Sex abuse: Being taken advantage of, or taking advantage of someone, sexually

Sex education: A lifetime study of sex information

Sex life: What you have plenty of time for after you graduate from school

"Spanking the monkey": Masturbation for boys

Sperm: In male semen; fertilizes the female's egg

Spermicides: Chemical foams and creams put into the vagina to try to prevent pregnancy and disease

Sponge: Contraceptive-filled; put into the vagina before sex to prevent pregnancy (presently off the market, but planned for reintroduction)

Statistic: What you don't want to be!

STD: Sexually Transmitted Disease

Sterilization: Operation to be made permanently unable to get, or get someone pregnant

"Stirring the soup": Masturbation for girls

Syphilis: A sex disease

Tampons: Thumb-size piece of cotton worn in the vagina to catch the blood from a period

Testicles: The male reproductive organs inside the scrotum which hang on each side of the penis

Time: What you have lots of—when it comes to sex

Toxic shock syndrome: Rare but serious medical problem that can come from using very absorbent tampons

Transsexual: Person who has the physical sex organs of one sex, but emotionally is the opposite sex

Transvestite: Person of one sex who likes to dress up like the opposite sex; usually men who like to wear women's clothes

Trust: Something or someone you can count on

Unfair: What it seems like life is sometimes

Urethra: Opening you urinate from

Uterus: Place in female where baby grows until it is born

Vagina: Opening between girl's legs that goes to the uterus

Vaginitis: Infection of the vagina

Vasectomy: Sterilization of the male by cutting the tiny tubes that sperm goes through

VD (venereal disease): Diseases gotten through sex activities

Venereal warts: Contagious bumps on the genitals

Virgin: A boy or girl who has never had sex

Vulva: The outside parts of the female genitals

Wet Dream: Ejaculation during sleep

Withdrawal: Trying to take the penis out of the vagina before any sperm gets into the vagina

You: The most important person in the world

Youth Clinics: Places you can call or visit and get good information and sexual advice from nurses and doctors who won't fuss at you

Zits: Slang word for acne, pimples, eczema, or other bumps you get on your face, usually before a date!

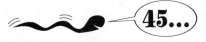 45...

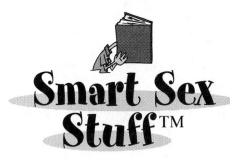

Smart Sex Stuff™

Carole Marsh's Original "Smart Sex Stuff" for Kids 7 - 17

THE 25 MOST ASKED QUESTIONS ABOUT SEX:
Questions Kids Ask Parents and Teachers Today...and the Honest Answers!

AIDS-ZITS: A 'SEXTIONARY' FOR KIDS 7-17/Excellent resource

THE BABY GAME/Any number can play; is not a board game/Each player has a baby and "cards" give instructions on what to do for it. Very humorous + points out consequences of parenthood!

(FIRST) AIDS: FRANK FACTS FOR KIDS/
In plain English for all ages

"Hello In There!": POETRY TO READ TO THE UNBORN BABY/EXCELLENT!

MY LIFETIME OF SEXUALITY TIMELINE

"NINE MONTHS IN MY MOMMY": AN AUTOBIOGRAPHY/
Fictional first-person autobiography gives kids respect for unborn child/KIDS WILL NEVER TAKE LIFE LIGHTLY AGAIN!

A PERIOD IS MORE THAN A PUNCTUATION MARK/
Especially for girls

"SEX ED": A Scrapbook of Sex Stuff for Curious Kids Who Have Questions, Want Answers!

SEX STUFF FOR KIDS: A Book of Practical Information & Ideas for Kids 7-17 & Their Parents & Teachers/Straight Stuff/Girl Stuff/Boy Stuff/Hot Stuff/Serious Stuff & Smart Stuff + the latest facts on AIDS/Illustrated/Glossary/Index

SPERM, SQUIRM & OTHER SQUIGGLY STUFF/Especially for boys

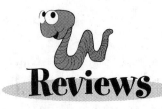

Reviews

Recommended for all public libraries.—Susan McBride/**Library Journal**

Addresses **all the questions and misconceptions** children have in plain language, interspersed with humor. Includes information about AIDS.—**Planned Parenthood LINKLINE**

Simply written for *today's* school children—about their body changes and how to learn about sex the <u>safe way</u>.—Josephine Hookway, R.N., OB-GYN, N.P.

A RICH RESOURCE—**a must** for parents! Clearly stated, sensible, and an effective combination of humor and seriousness. Kids *can* be sex smart.—L. Chennault, Teacher of the Year

Valuable additions to personal, community or academic library sex ed inventories.—Jim Cox Midwest Book Review

A MUST acquisition for parents, teachers, libraries, para-professionals, as well as the kids themselves—Diane Donovan, Book Reviewer, San Francisco, CA

Adolescents not ready to engage in sexual intimacy will find lots of support—Ann Barrett, Education Outreach Coordinator, Planned Parenthood Toronto *(in the SIECCAN Newsletter)*

Help us help kids be sex safe & sex smart! Thank you!

46...

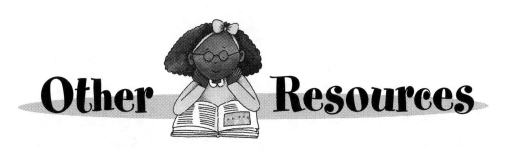

Other Resources

- Sexuality Information and Education Council of the US (SEICUS)
  www.seicus.org

- Planned Parenthood Federation of America
  www.plannedparenthood.org

- Planned Parenthood Health Centers—Online source for Reproductive Health Information
  www.plannedparenthood.org/ZIP.HTM

- Planned Parenthood/teenwire
  www.teenwire.com

- Centers for Disease Control and Prevention
  www.cdc.gov

- The National Campaign to Prevent Teen Pregnancy
  www.teenpregnancy.org

- www.webmd.com

- Children of the Night – Van Nuys, California
  Rescuing America's children from the ravages of street prostitution
  www.childrenofthenight.org

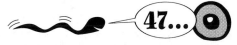

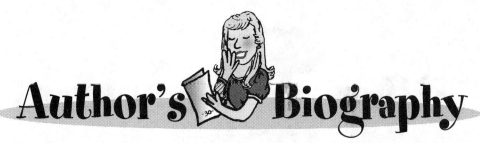

Author's Biography

Carole Marsh is the author of more than 36 books and other products on sex education for adults and children. Named 1979 Communicator of the Year by the Carolinas Association of Business communicators, she has spent a 25+ year career crafting fiction and non-fiction on all types of subjects for the 7-14-year old reader.

Marsh's sex education titles have been widely used in public and private schools, orphanages, church libraries, by Planned Parenthoods, and many other groups actively seeking to help young people. Her books have received outstanding reviews and recommendations all across the nation.

In 1980, Marsh was the keynote speaker at an important sex education forum held in Buffalo, New York. Recent media appearances include a discussion of her latest *The 25 Most Asked Questions About Sex: Questions Kids Ask Parents and Teachers Today…and the Honest Answers* on NBC's "Men are from Mars/Women are from Venus."

Marsh is a native of Marietta, Georgia. She is CEO of Gallopade International, Carole Marsh Family CD-ROMs, and onemillionactivities.com. She lives in Peachtree City, Georgia with her husband, Bob Longmeyer.

Parents and teachers, we'd love to hear from you! Let us know of any additional questions kids have asked you about sex. Complete this convenient postcard and drop it in the mail, or fax it to Gallopade International at 770/631-4810.

Dear Carole Marsh:

Kids have asked these questions about sex:

1.

2.

3.

Please include them in your next sex-ed book!

FROM:

Put Stamp Here

TO:
Carole Marsh
c/o Gallopade International
665 Hwy 74 South, Suite 600
Peachtree City, GA 30269
USA

48...